YOUR KNOWLEDGE HAS VALUE

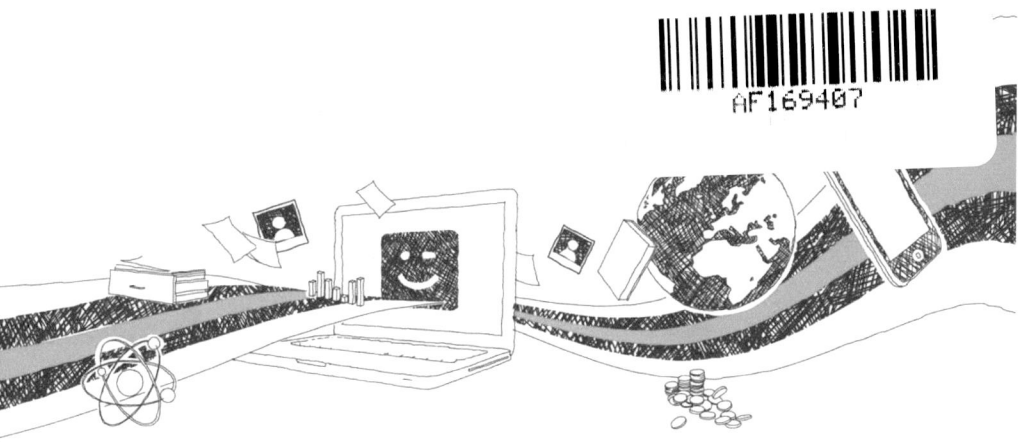

- We will publish your bachelor's and master's thesis, essays and papers

- Your own eBook and book - sold worldwide in all relevant shops

- Earn money with each sale

Upload your text at www.GRIN.com
and publish for free

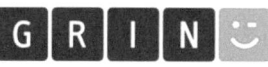

Bibliographic information published by the German National Library:

The German National Library lists this publication in the National Bibliography; detailed bibliographic data are available on the Internet at http://dnb.dnb.de .

This book is copyright material and must not be copied, reproduced, transferred, distributed, leased, licensed or publicly performed or used in any way except as specifically permitted in writing by the publishers, as allowed under the terms and conditions under which it was purchased or as strictly permitted by applicable copyright law. Any unauthorized distribution or use of this text may be a direct infringement of the author s and publisher s rights and those responsible may be liable in law accordingly.

Imprint:

Copyright © 2016 GRIN Verlag, Open Publishing GmbH
Print and binding: Books on Demand GmbH, Norderstedt Germany
ISBN: 9783668575295

This book at GRIN:

http://www.grin.com/en/e-book/381312/psychology-of-cystic-fibrosis

Patrick Kimuyu

Psychology of Cystic Fibrosis

GRIN Publishing

GRIN - Your knowledge has value

Since its foundation in 1998, GRIN has specialized in publishing academic texts by students, college teachers and other academics as e-book and printed book. The website www.grin.com is an ideal platform for presenting term papers, final papers, scientific essays, dissertations and specialist books.

Visit us on the internet:

http://www.grin.com/

http://www.facebook.com/grincom

http://www.twitter.com/grin_com

Psychology of Cystic Fibrosis

Patrick K. Kimuyu

Psychology of Cystic Fibrosis

Scientists define cystic fibrosis (CF) as an autosomal recessive genetic disorder affecting lungs, but can also progress to intestine, pancreas and liver. Since the disorder mostly affects lungs, the affected patients have difficulties in breathing. The disorder affects more than 30,000 people in the United States. In 2011, 309 people suffered from cystic fibrosis in Western Australia. The median age of death for people suffering from CF was reported as 27 years. 60% of CF deaths are attributed to pulmonary complications (Department of Health, Western Australia, 2013, p. 9). However, CF patients can live more than forty years with proper care and medication. According to the Department of Health, Western Australia (2013, p. 9), more adult people suffered from CF compared to children in western Australian in the 2010. Scientists believe that CF is caused by many gene mutations for the protein cystic fibrosis transmembrane conductance regulator (CFTR). Precisely, this protein is essential in regulating components of digestive fluids, mucus and sweat (Griffiths et al, 2004, p. 453). Majority of health people have two copies of the CFTR gene while carriers have only one working copy. Evidently, people suffering from the CF have no working copy of CFTR gene. The disorder is associated with many gastrointestinal complications which, include biliary cirrhosis, intestine obstruction and bile duct proliferation (Rapee, Schniering & Hudson, 2009, p. 339).

Children suspected to suffer from CF should be diagnosed by carrying out sweat test. However, this procedure can be delayed to allow infants sweat gland produce enough sweat. The development of newborn screening has allowed more children suffering from CF get early diagnosis hence reducing hospitalization (Cruz et al, 2009, p. 572).

Seemingly, human development is one of the most complex areas in the field of psychology. Many changes occur in human beings during the course of their lives. Developmental psychology tries to interlinks stages that involve gradual accumulation of knowledge, innate mental structures and learning in human life. According to Erikson's model on stages of psychosocial development, human beings pass through eight stages from infancy to adulthood. During each stage of development, a person meets and masters new challenges. Additionally, each stage is built on successful completion of the prior stages (Jane, 2012, p. 8). Failure to complete each stage of development can give rise to problems during future stages. The development of the eight stages is influenced by both the biological and socio-cultural forces.

Notably, the bonding relationship between the infant and parent is often based on their mutual connection of their dyad. Psychologist argues that both the child and parent mental representation are involved in the attachment process. Ideally, the parent-child relationship is essential for the developing infant (Cruz et al, 2009, p. 573). The quality of attachment determines the child psychological factors such as behavior regulation, emotions, social skills and the ability to manage stressful conditions. Parental distress affects the attachment, which often coincide with the timing for the CF diagnosis. Due to the emotional nature of CF diagnosis, some parents become hypervigilance making misinterpretation of common behaviors as signs of CF (Rapee, Schniering & Hudson, 2009, p. 338). This complicates the parent-child relationship leading to maladaptive attachment. Research has found out that infants with maladaptive attachment have low BMI and poor nutritional status.

The first phase of development (Trust vs. Mistrust) is the most fundamental in the life of a child. Since the child is dependent entirely on caregivers, the quality and dependability of such people are vital in their development. Children who develop trust of their caregiver will feel safe and secure in the world. Due to cystic fibrosis, some caregivers might become emotionally unavailable, inconsistent hence contributing the development of mistrust in their children. Such children will grow with a feeling that the world is fearful and unpredictable place for human beings. Additionally, failure for caregivers to attend conditions such as belly pain, bloating and pulmonary insufficient will increase mistrust (Melamed et al, 2013, p. 18).

Researchers also argue that the second phase of development (Toddler -- Age 1 to 2) might delay due to cystic fibrosis. Normally, a child develops a sense of autonomy during the toddler phase. They learn how to talk, use the toilet, walk and carry out activities on their own. Parents and caregiver should encourage their children initiative and correct them whenever they make mistakes. However, if parents become overactive to such children owing top stress emanating from their medication, diet requirement and general wellbeing, such children will begin to feel ashamed of their initiative and doubt their capabilities (Melamed et al, 2013, p. 29).

During early childhood (Age 2 to 5), children become more engaged in social interaction with people around them. The rate of motor skills development is also high making them active. Children also learn to control their fantasies, eagerness and responsibilities. Parents should encourage their children about right discipline and accept guiltiness. However, due to special treatment accorded to children suffering from cystic fibrosis, it might become difficult in instilling the right discipline them. Additionally, encouraging such children to be independent is hard since they require constant attention of caregivers. The burden of treatment even during when the child has mild disease can lead to conflicts. The child might develop a feeling that his/her parents are harsh (Jane, 2012, p. 8).

Children learn social relationships during the adolescence stage (12 to 18 years). During this stage, teens develop a sense of personal and self-identity. Success makes teen stay true to themselves while failure leads to confusion. More importantly, coping with relationships and cystic fibrosis is becomes challenging to the affected teenagers. Some teenagers might face barrier to forming relationships such as embarrassment due to symptoms or lack of independence. Additionally, symptoms of cystic fibrosis become severe during human development making the affected teenager remain under watchful eye of their relatives. This affects their social lives and relationships. Losing a friend who also has cystic fibrosis is a hard pie to swallow (Sauter, Heyne & Westenberg, 2009, p. 312). Such situation increase fear and distress to the affected teenagers.

Many CF adolescent have concerns on how their condition will affect their lives. Some wonder whether they will ever finish school, get jobs, partners and starts families. Other tend to reduce the number of friends especially of the opposite sex since they believe their condition require sensitive attention. The symptoms produced by CF are embarrassing and distressing. Research also indicates that gastrointestinal symptoms make many adolescents miss school and social activities due to embarrassment (Iles & Lowton, 2008, p. 437). Doing chest physiotherapy and taking pancreatic enzymes in the front of peers have a negative impact on patients.

According to Erikson's model, the virtues learned during the age of six are competence. It is vital to note that fundamentals of play and technology are developed during this age. Children who lose hope of an industrious association are pulled back to lives of isolation leading to the development of less conscious familial rivalry as seen in CF (Sauter, Heyne & Westenberg, 2009, p. 315).

Since cystic fibrosis is a progressive disorder, the burden that comes with the symptoms and treatment are stressful to both the child and his/her family. Multiple pain locations are common to CF patients, and this affects their quality of life. CF patients have to use medications to fight chest pain. Additionally, the treatment and cost of medicine required for the patient to live longer are expensive hence increasing stressful condition to one's family (Wong & Heriot, 2008, p. 352). The nature and treatment required may interfere with day to day life of both the child and his/her family.

It is also vital to note that the demands of undergoing procedures such as cough swabs, feeding and blood tests are usually tough for children. This issue is the fundamental source of behavioral challenge faced by relatives with children suffering from cystic fibrosis. Ideally, as children with cystic fibrosis grow, they became capable of enjoying the same experiences, threats and opportunities just like their peers. However, the feeling of being different from other is understandable especially in school settings. This problem is compounded by awkward treatment regime and special diet (Rapee, Schniering & Hudson, 2009, p. 317). Researchers also indicate that causes of bullying are common to children suffering from cystic fibrosis since they are smaller, and thinner compared to their peers.

Psychologists also assert that the feeling of independence and responsibility towards medication can cause frustration to people with cystic fibrosis. The desire to be like other people can lead to teenagers neglecting their treatment hence worsening the symptoms. Further, teenagers with cystic fibrosis suffer from lack of control to certain aspect of their own lives and feeling of uncertainty leading to anxiety, depression and insecurity (Rapee, Schniering & Hudson, 2009, p. 321).

The body image of people with cystic fibrosis varies from that of the other people. For instance, the onset of the period is delayed by one or two years during the puberty stage with consequent stature. Biologically, CF delays the release of gonadotrophin releasing hormone from the hypothalamus (Sauter, Heyne & Westenberg, 2009, p. 319). Other symptoms that are specific to children suffering from cystic fibrosis include; delayed growth, failure to gain weight due to the increasing catabolic rate, weight loss resulting from poor absorption and production of calorie dense sputum, clubbed fingers. Researchers believe that vas deferens is absent in 98% of men suffering from cystic fibrosis. As a result, seminal vesicles of such men become dysfunctional resulting to low ejaculate volume. These symptoms have been found to increase emotional distress to the affected patients. The increasing number of chest infections and flare up can keep teenagers out of school for a long period making it harder to cope with other both socially and academically.

Children at age of six become aware of themselves as human beings hence work hard in becoming good and responsible individuals. Age of six is also marked with the development of reasoning cooperation skills. Psychologists also argue that children at the age of six become capable of grasping the concept of time and space in more practical and logical manner (Wong & Heriot, 2008, p. 351).CF condition affects growth compromising their development.

The age of six is also marked with the eagerness to learn and grasping of more complex skills such as telling time, reading and writing. Moral values and the recognition of individual and cultural differences becomes vital stage during the age of six. They also start to groom with little assistance (Casier et al, 2008, p. 635). Majority of CF patients require attention of caregivers.

The elementary school period is vital for helping the development of self-confidence in children. Children at this age work hard in an effort to draw attention and recognition from parents, teachers and peers. They draw pictures, write sentences on their own and solves additional problem. Encouraging children to do such thing a praising their efforts help in sharpening their diligent skills. Children unable of completing such task owing to CF condition develop feeling of inferiority about their capabilities. Further, children will start to pursue their dreams by either joining sports or playing music during the age of six (Casier et al, 2008, p. 71). Failure to encourage children develop their interest during this time may lead to lack of motivation, lethargy and low self-esteem.

According to Szyndlera et al (2005, p.131), 15-20% of the young people in Australia suffer from a psychiatric disorder due to depression. This percentage has reduced compared to a decade ago. Newborn babies are screened for CF and parent given the necessary support making them raise their children more effectively. Currently, families and children with CF are able to access ethos of the clinic continuity of care from a physician with good nursing psychosocial support. During the adolescent period, teens require great independence in contrast to their condition. Monitoring and parental involvement is critical for good adherence of medication. More importantly, parental availability, low family stress and integrative family coping can lead to better health outcomes.

Though research indicate that chronically ill patients engage in risky activities such as binge drinking, smoking and unprotected sex compared to their healthy counterpart, youths with CF demonstrates less of such behaviors. However, more than 20% of youths suffering from CF smoke tobacco, a concerning statistics due to the implications of smoking to pulmonary function and nutrition. Normally, many youths develop eating disorders during adolescent, and this raises concern about CF due to relationships between mortality and nutritional status (Casier et al, 2008, p. 69).

It is vital to note that receiving initial diagnosis results that a child or loved member of the family has cystic fibrosis comes with a huge shock. During this condition, people experience a wide range of emotions such as anger, guiltiness and denial. Denial and anger can affect one's day to day activities as they spend their time meditating on the next step of their lives. Further, raising a child with a medical condition to lead a normal live and preparing them to enter the adult world is one of the most challenging tasks to carry out. Children suffering from cystic fibrosis suffer from many challenges, which require both emotional and material support. Due to this support, children without cystic fibrosis might feel neglected (Bryon, Shearer & Davies, 2008, p. 635). Evidently, some parents try addressing and focusing their attention to cystic fibrosis child leaving other children with a feeling of alienation.

As a future health care professional, understanding human development and psychological responses to illness will be vital in helping spread CF awareness and develop better coping measures. The management of CF among adolescent has been a stumbling block in the last couple of years. Educating adolescents and their families about the disease and its treatment can aid in reducing the mortality rate (Jane, 2012, p. 9). Additionally, I will educate the affected teenagers and their families on methods of coping with stress. Evidently, emotional distress is the leading cause of lack of adherence to medication due to the secondary denial of the illness. Many adolescent fails to see the future consequences of their actions and end up prioritizing their social lives ahead of illness. Lack of adherence among adolescent can be due to a poor family and social networks, chaotic home life and cultural beliefs. As a future health professional, I will link up with other professional in availing support to the affected people (Jane, 2012, p. 10).

As a future health care professional, I will ensure that diagnostic tests are accorded more privacy and confidentiality especially when dealing with adolescents. Additionally, improving communication with adolescents will help in fighting their stress (Segal, 2008, p. 11). I will also help patients in managing their stress, fears and phobia. This can be done by showing the patients' and their families that CF is manageable condition only through appropriate medication, gene therapy, lung transplantation and surgery for newborns. Notably parental testing is also vital in reducing chances of CF in their off springs (Wong & Heriot, 2008, p. 350).

Since infertility is one of the major challenges affecting people suffering from cystic fibrosis, I will encourage them to get children through assisted reproductive techniques. Additionally, maintenance lung health is essential in the treatment of CF. As a health care professional, I will encourage affected patients to go for airway clearance treatment. I will also advocate for gastrointestinal treatment measures such as pancreatic enzyme replacement and vitamins, high caloric intake of dietary supplements (Bennett et al, 2008, p. 290).

As a health professional, I will help parents in implementing developmentally-appropriate effective routines around both CF-specific treatment tasks and general daily activities capable of promoting positive reciprocal relationships. I will also try to solicit for resources from both the government and non-governmental agencies in order to develop a CF platform. The platform will have the mandate of interacting with affected patients and families and sharing their concerns and worries. Funds obtained from the supporting bodies will also be used to sponsor and support medical treatment of needy patients (Department of Health, Western Australia, 2013, p. 14).

In conclusion, cystic fibrosis refers to an autosomal recessive disorder affecting lungs leading to difficulties in breathing. The disease affects more than 30,000 people in the United States. In 2011, 309 people were suffering from cystic fibrosis in Western Australia. Out of this number, 60% succumbs to lungs related complications. This disorder can also lead to gastrointestinal complications such as bile duct proliferation, intestinal blockage and biliary problems.

Human development is one of the complex processes in the field of psychology. Human development interlinks various stages ranging from the development of mental structures, cognitive skills and the learning process. According to Erikson's theory, human development involves eight core stages. The success of the progressive stage is affected by the previous stage. The attachment process between parents and children during infancy is vital for effective development of behavior, emotions and social skills. Since cystic fibrosis requires constant attention during infancy, some parents may become overactive to their children affecting the attachment process. Cystic fibrosis also slows down growth and development. This can affect activities such as walking, talking and been basic skills especially during the second stage of development. The age of five is vital in the development of social skills. Children suffering from cystic fibrosis might have difficulties in socializing with their peers since they require constant medical attention. Additionally, children suffering from cystic fibrosis are pulled back from the industrious association leading to the development of less conscious familial rivalry.

Cystic fibrosis affects adolescents since they find it hard in forming relationships owing to embarrassment of symptoms. Such youths have a constant worry on their lives, educations and jobs. Some youths reduce the number of their friends especially of the opposite sex due to the sensitivity if cystic fibrosis. Their families and relatives also suffer distress and emotional torture. Medication involved in managing cystic fibrosis is too high for some families to afford, and this increases their stress. As a future health care professional, I will prioritize awareness campaigns and education in the society. I will also form a platform capable of soliciting funds for supporting the affected families. I will also carry out dose adherence campaigns

References

Griffiths, L et al. 2004. Cystic fibrosis patients and families support cross-infection measures. *European Respiratory Journal.* 24(3):449–452.

Sauter, M, Heyne D & Westenberg M. 2009. Cognitive behavior therapy for anxious adolescents: developmental influences on treatment design and delivery. *Clin Child Fam Psychol Rev*;12(4):310–335.

Casier, A, et al. 2008. The role of acceptance in psychological functioning in adolescents with cystic fibrosis: a preliminary study. *Psychology and Health*.23(5):629–638.

Bryon, M, Shearer J & Davies H. 2008. Eating disorders and disturbance in children and adolescents with cystic fibrosis. *Children's Health Care.* 37(1):67–77.

Iles, N & Lowton K. 2008. Young people with cystic fibrosis' concerns for their future: when and how should concerns be addressed, and by whom? *J Interprof Care.* 22(4):436–438

Rapee, M, Schniering, A & Hudson, L. 2009. Anxiety disorders during childhood and adolescence: origins and treatment. *Annu. Rev. Clin. Psychol.* 5:311–341.

Bennett, D et al. 2008. Monitoring and internalizing symptoms among youths with cystic fibrosis. *Children's Health Care.* 37(4):278–292.

Cruz, I, et al. 2009. Anxiety and depression in cystic fibrosis. *Semin Respir Crit Care Med.* 30(5):569–578.

Wong, G & Heriot, A. 2008. Parents of children with cystic fibrosis: how they hope, cope and despair. *Child Care Health Dev.* 34(3):344–354.

Segal, Y. 2008. Adolescence: what the cystic fibrosis team needs to know. *Journal of the Royal Society of Medicine*,101 Suppl 1, 15-27.

Szyndlera, E et al. 2005. Psychological and family functioning and quality of life in adolescents with cystic fibrosis. *Journal of Cystic Fibrosis,* 4,135-144.

Melamed, B et al. 2013. *Child Health Psychology.* Plymouth: Psychology Press.

Jane, O. 2012. *Health Psychology: A Textbook: A textbook Open University Press.* New York City: McGraw-Hill International.

Department of Health, Western Australia. 2013. WA Cystic Fibrosis Model of Care. [Online] Available at: http://www.healthnetworks.health.wa.gov.au/modelsofcare/docs/CF_Model_of_Care.pdf [Accessed on 24th September 2014].

YOUR KNOWLEDGE HAS VALUE

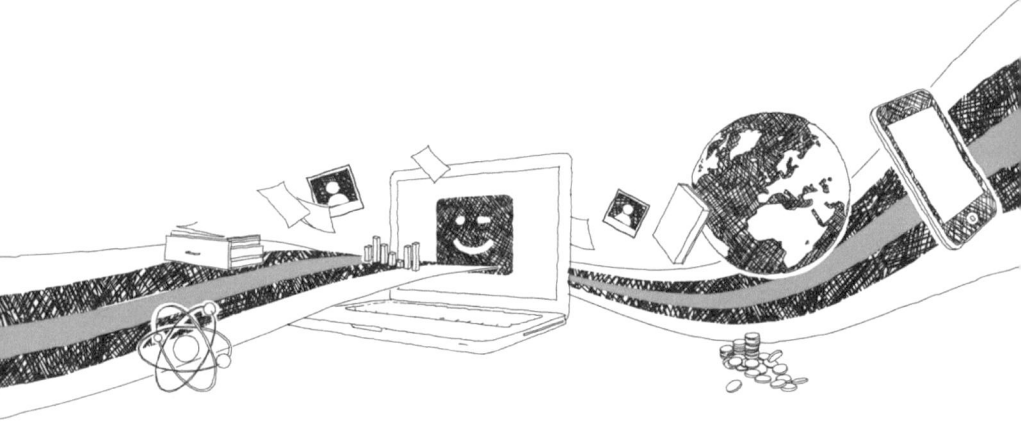

- We will publish your bachelor's and master's thesis, essays and papers

- Your own eBook and book - sold worldwide in all relevant shops

- Earn money with each sale

Upload your text at www.GRIN.com
and publish for free

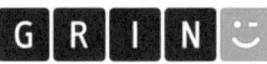